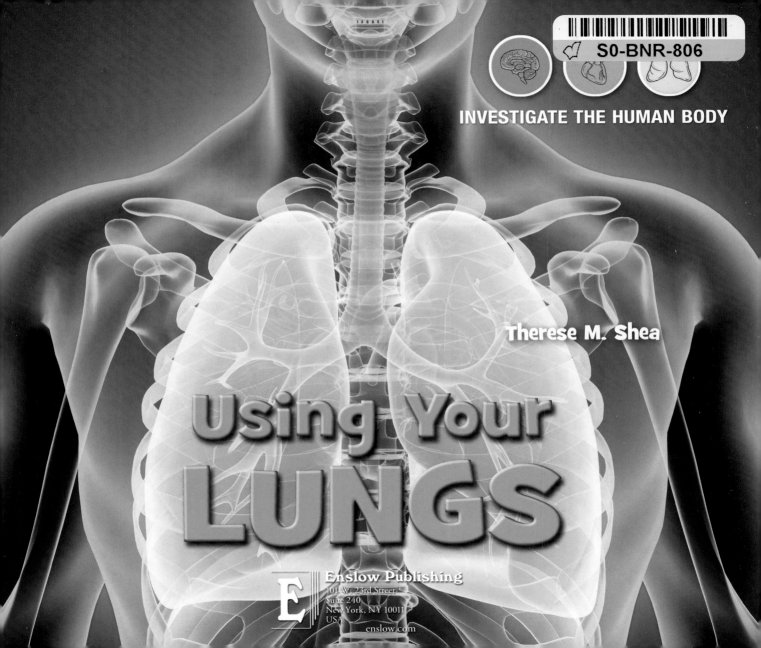

INVESTIGATE THE HUMAN BODY

Therese M. Shea

Using Your LUNGS

Enslow Publishing
101 W. 23rd Street
Suite 240
New York, NY 10011
USA
enslow.com

S0-BNR-806

●●○ Words to Know

bacteria Tiny creatures that can only be seen with a microscope.

blood vessel A small tube that carries blood to different parts of a person's body.

cell The smallest basic part of a living thing.

cough To force air through your throat with a short, loud noise.

muscle One of the parts of the body that allow movement.

organ A part of the body that has a certain job.

relax To become less tight.

sac A part inside the body that is shaped like a bag. It usually contains liquid or air.

tumor A lump found in or on the body that is made up of unusual cells.

water vapor A gas form of water.

Contents

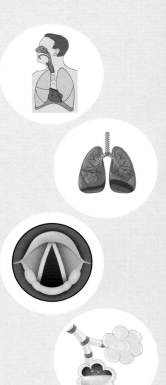

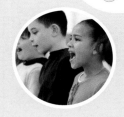

Just Breathe!

Oxygen is a gas in the air that every person and animal needs to live. It's easy to get oxygen. Just breathe! Your body has special **organs** for breathing. They're called the lungs.

Lungs in Action

The human body has two lungs. Each lung looks a bit like a bag. One is on each side of your chest. The one on the left is a little smaller.

The lungs rest on a sheet of **muscle** called the diaphragm. When the diaphragm contracts, or tightens, the lungs grow larger. Air fills them. Muscles lift the ribs up and out to give the lungs room.

When you breathe out, or exhale, your diaphragm **relaxes** and moves up. The rib muscles also relax. Air is then forced out of the lungs.

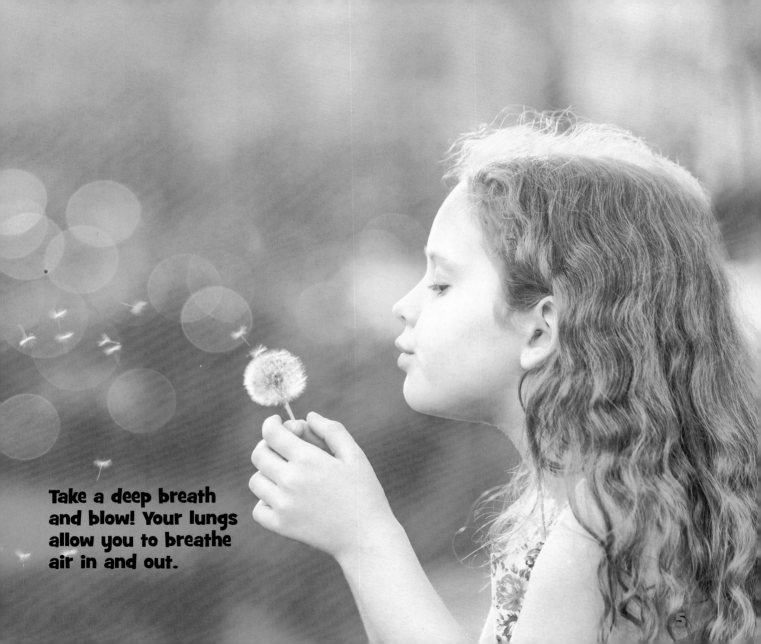

Take a deep breath and blow! Your lungs allow you to breathe air in and out.

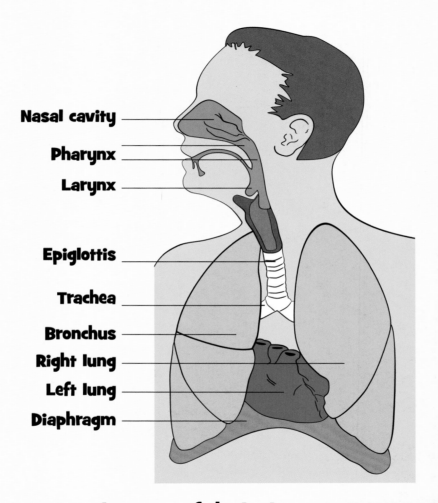

Nasal cavity

Pharynx

Larynx

Epiglottis

Trachea

Bronchus

Right lung

Left lung

Diaphragm

The lungs are a key part of the body's respiratory system.

Why Do I Hiccup?

Hiccups happen when the diaphragm tightens quickly a number of times. This may mean the stomach is bothered by something.

Respiration

The air that goes into your lungs contains oxygen. Every **cell** in your body needs this gas for energy. The air that goes out of your lungs contains the gas carbon dioxide. This is a waste that your cells need to get rid of.

The act of taking in oxygen and letting go of carbon dioxide is called respiration. All the body parts that make this happen are called the respiratory system. The brain is in charge of the respiratory system.

Inside the Lungs

You probably don't think too much about breathing. But a lot of things happen in your body with each breath you take. Let's follow a breath of air into the human body and find out how oxygen gets to your cells. It's a bit like a maze!

Breathing In

When you breathe in through your nose or mouth, the air goes in a tube called the trachea, or windpipe. The trachea connects to two tubes called the bronchi. The bronchi lead to smaller tubes in the lungs called bronchioles. The bronchioles connect to tiny **sacs** called alveoli.

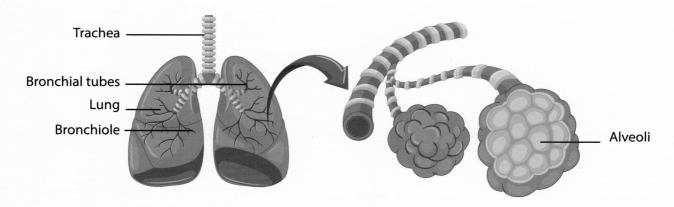

Air travels through the trachea, bronchi, bronchiole, and alveoli, allowing oxygen to reach all parts of your body.

The alveoli are covered by **blood vessels** called capillaries. They carry blood that needs oxygen. The oxygen you breathe in passes through the thin walls of the alveoli and enters the blood. Blood with oxygen then goes to the heart. From there, the blood can be pumped to all the cells in the body.

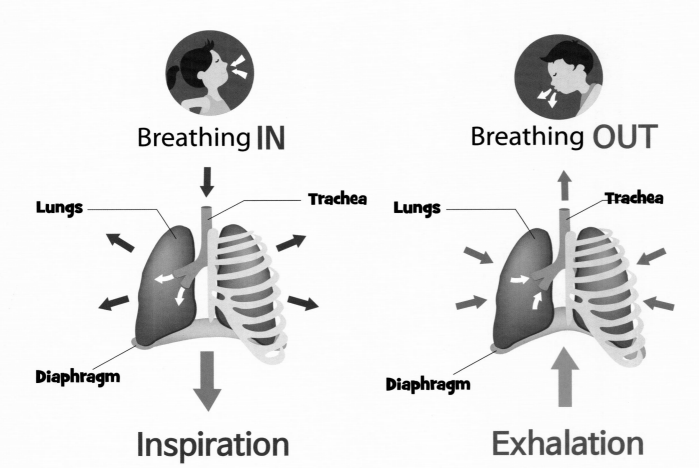

Breathing IN

Breathing OUT

Lungs

Trachea

Diaphragm

Lungs

Trachea

Diaphragm

Inspiration

Exhalation

The body takes in oxygen when you inhale and releases carbon dioxide when you exhale.

Inside the Lungs

The lungs contain about 60,000 bronchioles and about 600 million alveoli!

Breathing Out

The blood traveling to the lungs gets rid of waste at the same time it's getting oxygen. The waste includes carbon dioxide and **water vapor**. The waste air leaves the alveoli and goes out through the bronchioles, the bronchi, and the trachea. You finally let the air out through your mouth and nose.

The lungs also trap harmful things that come in with air. The lungs are lined with a sticky matter called mucus. **Bacteria**, dust, and other bits stick to the mucus. You may breathe or **cough** these things out.

Beautiful Breath

Babies breathe up to 44 times a minute. Adults breathe about 16 times a minute. When people are asleep, they breathe more slowly. You can make yourself breathe differently by thinking about it. However, usually your brain makes you breathe the amount you should.

More Breath, More Oxygen

Your brain changes how quickly you breathe sometimes. When you run around, your cells take in more oxygen and give out more carbon dioxide. So, your body needs to breathe more to take in more oxygen and get rid of more carbon dioxide. You may breathe up to 60 times a minute.

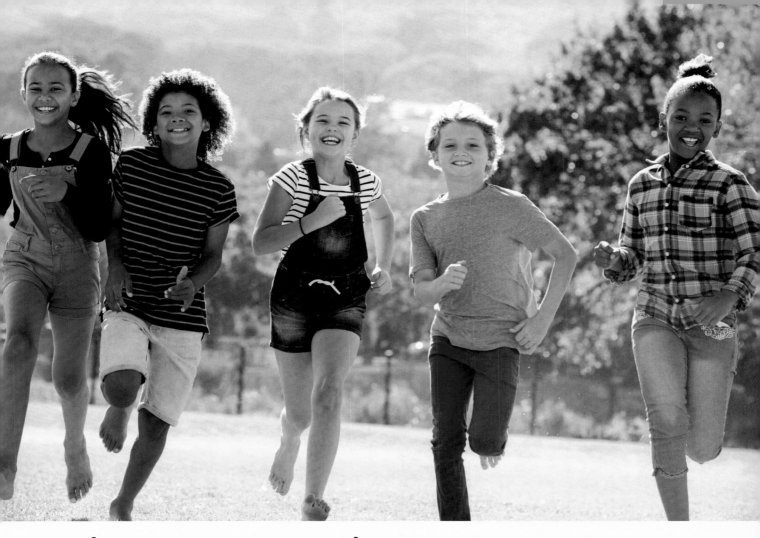

When you are active, you breathe more quickly so your body gets more oxygen.

Get Moving

When you exercise, blood moves more quickly through your blood vessels to get oxygen where it's needed.

Your brain might also make you breathe more quickly if you feel nervous or worried. That's because your brain is getting your body ready to move fast if it needs to.

Let's Talk

You also need breath when you talk, laugh, and sing. Above your trachea is a body part called the larynx, or the voice box. Across the top of the larynx are two folds called the vocal cords. Air from your lungs pushes through your closed vocal cords. This causes them to vibrate, or move back and forth. That makes sound!

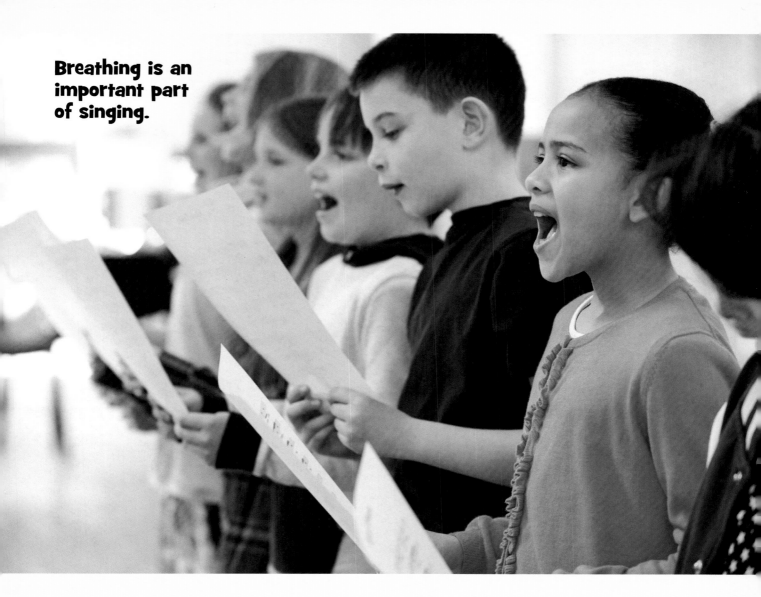

Breathing is an important part of singing.

Larynx

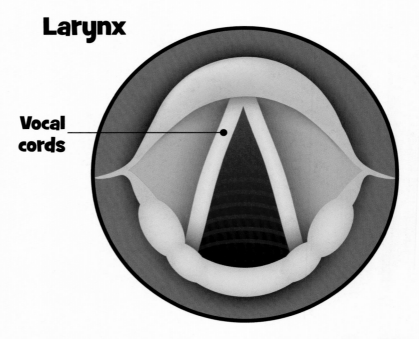

Vocal cords

Your vocal cords vibrate when air passes through. This allows you to speak and sing.

The more air that comes out of your larynx, the louder and longer the sound you make. Your tongue, teeth, lips, jaw, and the roof of your mouth help shape sounds into words people can understand.

Lung Health

When our lungs are healthy, we don't even think about them. But sometimes we can't breathe easily, cough a lot, or feel pain in our chest. This might mean that something is wrong with the lungs. Most sicknesses that affect our lungs pass quickly. However, some are more serious.

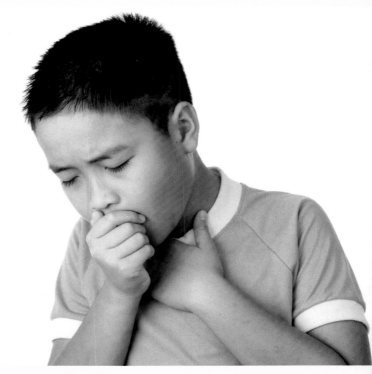

Sometimes lung problems cause us to cough or have a hard time breathing.

Lung Problems

Tuberculosis is a serious lung disease, or illness, caused by harmful bacteria. It can cause holes in the lungs. Another lung disease is pneumonia. It's caused by a virus or bacteria. It stops the alveoli from working well.

Emphysema is a disease in which the walls of the alveoli break. Sometimes harmful **tumors** can grow in the lungs. This is called lung cancer.

Pretty in Pink
Healthy lungs are a pink color. Lungs with emphysema can appear brown.

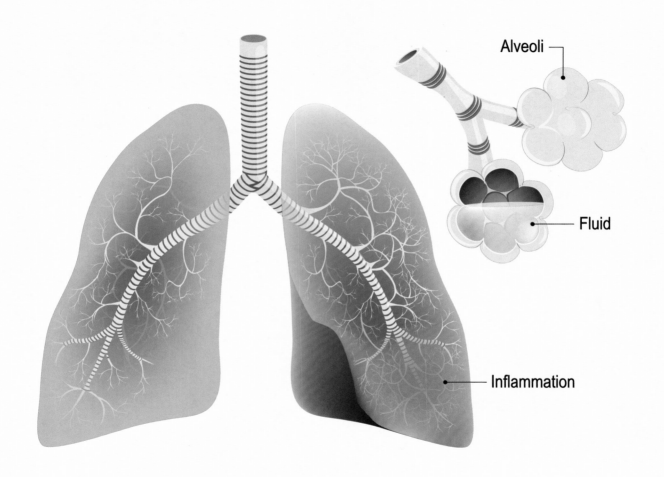

Alveoli

Fluid

Inflammation

Pneumonia is a disease that occurs when fluid gets in the alveoli. This makes it hard to breathe.

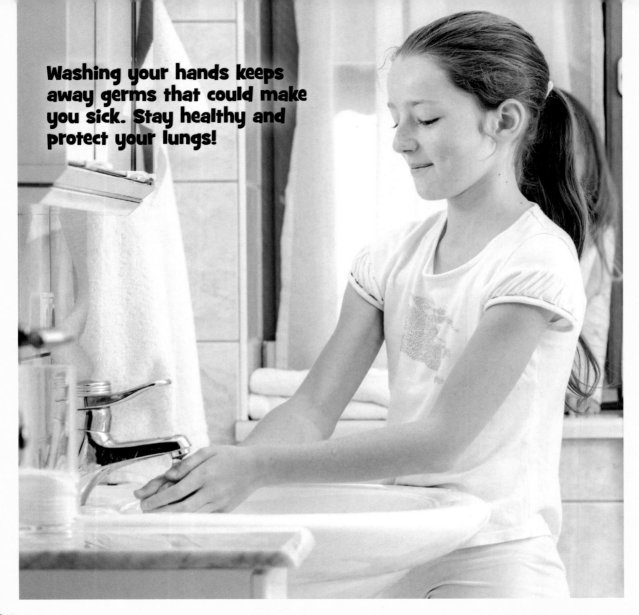

Washing your hands keeps away germs that could make you sick. Stay healthy and protect your lungs!

Smoking is one of the main causes of emphysema and lung cancer. One way to keep your lungs healthy is to never smoke. It's also important to stay away from others who smoke. The smoke others breathe out is called secondhand smoke. It can be just as dangerous to your lungs as smoking.

Love Your Lungs

You can avoid getting sick with the flu and other illnesses that can affect your lungs. The best way is by washing your hands often!

Another way to keep your lungs healthy is exercise. When you exercise, you breathe more deeply and take in more air. That makes your lungs become stronger and better at giving your body the oxygen it needs. So keep moving and breathing. Love your lungs!

Activity: Paper-Bag Lungs

●●● What You Need:

- 2 small paper bags
- 2 straws

- duct tape
- black marker

Step 1: Look at the picture of the inside of the lungs on page 9.

Step 2: Use the marker to draw bronchioles and alveoli on each paper bag.

Step 3: Open the bags. Place a straw a few inches inside each bag. These are your bronchi.

Step 4: Gather the top of the bag around the straw. Tape tightly.

Step 5: Blow into each straw to put air into your paper-bag lungs.

Step 6: Let the air out by squeezing the paper-bag lungs.

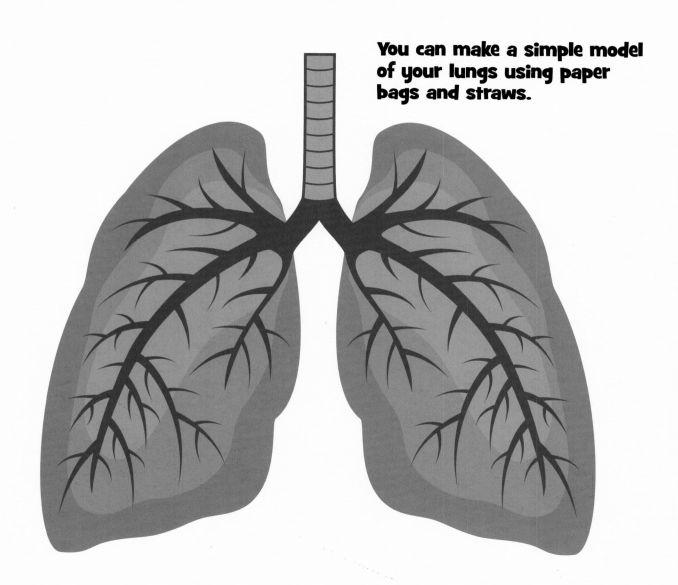

You can make a simple model of your lungs using paper bags and straws.

●●● Learn More

Books

Fittleworth, George. *Your Lungs*. New York, NY: Gareth Stevens Publishing, 2017.

Kenney, Karen. *Respiratory System*. Minneapolis, MN: Pogo, 2017.

Manolis, Kay. *The Respiratory System*. Minnetonka, MN: Bellwether Media, 2016.

Websites

Lungs
www.dkfindout.com/us/human-body/lungs-and-breathing/lungs/
Check out this fun, interactive website about how your lungs work.

Your Lungs & Respiratory System
kidshealth.org/en/kids/lungs.html
Learn more about these important body parts from a doctor.

●●● Index

Published in 2020 by Enslow Publishing, LLC
101 W. 23rd Street, Suite 240, New York, NY 10011

Library of Congress Cataloging-in-Publication Data
Names: Shea, Therese M., author.
Title: Using your lungs / Therese M. Shea.
Description: New York : Enslow Publishing, 2020. | Series: Investigate the human body | Includes bibliographical references and index. | Audience: Grades K-4.
Identifiers: LCCN 2019004897| ISBN 9781978512870 (library bound) | ISBN 9781978512856 (paperback) | ISBN 9781978512863 (6 pack)
Subjects: LCSH: Lungs--Juvenile literature.
Classification: LCC QM261 .S54 2020 | DDC 612.2/4--dc23
LC record available at https://lccn.loc.gov/2019004897

Printed in the United States of America

To Our Readers: We have done our best to make sure all website addresses in this book were active and appropriate when we went to press. However, the author and the publisher have no control over and assume no liability for the material available on those websites or on any websites they may link to. Any comments or suggestions can be sent by email to customerservice@enslow.com.

Photos Credits: Using Your Lungs – Research by Bruce Donnola Cover, p. 1 MDGRPHCS /Shutterstock.com; pp. 3, 6 udaix/ Shutterstock.com; pp. 3, 9 GraphicsRF/ Shutterstock.com; pp. 3, 16, 19 Designua/ Shutterstock.com; pp. 3, 15 SpeedKingz/Shutterstock.com; p. 5 Yuliya Evstratenko/ Shutterstock.com; p. 10 Jakinnboaz/ Shutterstock.com; p. 13 Monkey Business Images/ Shutterstock.com; p. 17 TinnaPong/ Shutterstock.com; p. 20 bonzodog/ Shutterstock.com; p. 23 freesoulproduction/ Shutterstock.com; cover graphics blackpencil/Shutterstock.com